KNOWLEDGE GUIDE TO
TENDINITIS

Essential Manual To Effective Treatments, Exercises, And Pain Management For Inflammation And Joint Health

DR. AARON BRANUM

Copyright © 2024 BY DR. AARON BRANUM

All rights reserved. Except for brief quotations embodied in critical reviews and certain other noncommercial uses permitted by copyright law, no part of this publication may be reproduced, distributed, or transmitted in any form or by any means, Including photocopying, recording, or other electronic or mechanical methods, without the prior written permission of the publisher.

Disclaimer:

The data in this book, is solely meant to be informative and instructional.

This book is not intended to replace expert medical advice, diagnosis, or care. No medical, health, or other professional services are offered by the author, publisher, or any affiliated parties

Individual outcomes may differ in the practice of these therapies, which entail a variety of approaches and methodologies.

A one-on-one session with a trained or certified healthcare professional is still preferable. It is best to consult a trained healthcare provider before making any decisions regarding your health.

The author of this book is not affiliated with any specific website, product, or organization related to any of these therapies.

All reasonable measures have been taken by the author and publisher to guarantee the authenticity and dependability of the material contained in this book

Contents

CHAPTER ONE 13
TENDONS' ANATOMY AND FUNCTION 13
- Examining The Tendon Structure 13
- Tendon Functions In The Body 14
- Tendons' Function In Movement 15
- Tendon Health Influencing Factors 16
- Tendon Strength And Flexibility Are Important 17

CHAPTER TWO 19
TYPES AND ETIOLOGY OF TENDINOPATHY .. 19
- Various Forms Of Tendinitis 19
- Finding The Root Causes 20
- Comprehending Incidental Elements 21
- Lifestyle's Effect On The Development Of Tendinitis 22
- Risk Elements Linked To Tendinitis 23

CHAPTER THREE 25
INDICATES AND SYMPTOMS 25
- Identifying Early Warning Indications 25
- Typical Symptoms 26

How The Affected Area Affects The
Symptoms 27
Recognising Acute Vs Chronic Tendinitis ... 29
When To Get Medical Help 31
CHAPTER FOUR 33
DIAGNOSIS AND EVALUATION 33
Synopsis Of Diagnostic Techniques 33
Methods Of Physical Examination 33
Imaging Examinations For Precise Diagnosis
.... 34
Speaking With Medical Experts 35
The Value Of A Thorough Evaluation 35
CHAPTER FIVE 37
OPTIONS FOR TREATMENT 37
Non-Surgical Methods Of Therapy 37
Painkillers 40
Methods Of Physical Treatment 42
Function Of Relaxation And Activity
Adjustment 45
Surgical Procedures In
More Serious Situations 47

CHAPTER SIX ... 51
PREVENTIVE ACTIONS ... 51
- The Value Of Preventive Techniques ... 51
- Including Appropriate Ergonomics ... 51
- Warm-Up And Cool-Down Techniques That Work ... 52
- Changes In Lifestyle To Lower Risk ... 53
- Encouraging General Tendon Health ... 53

CHAPTER SEVEN ... 55
RESTORATION AS WELL AS RECOVERY ... 55
- Knowing How The Recovery Process Works ... 55
- Exercises And Methods For Rehabilitation . 58
- Returning Gradually To The Activity Guidelines ... 60
- Handling Obstacles During Rehabilitation .. 62
- Long-Term Methods Of Recurrence Prevention ... 64

CHAPTER EIGHT ... 67
OPTIONAL THERAPIES ... 67
- Examining Complementary Medicine ... 67

Acupuncture's Function In Pain Management 68
Advantages Of Therapeutic Massage 69
Using Supports And Braces 70
Possibility Of Herbal Remedies Being Effective 70

CHAPTER NINE 73
COMMON QUESTIONS AND ANSWERS 73
Dispelling Myths Regarding Tendinitis 73
Handling The Fear And Anxiety Caused By The Illness 74
Faqs Regarding Changes In Lifestyle 75
Resolving Surgery-Related Fears 76
Sources Of Continued Assistance And Knowledge 77

ABOUT THIS BOOK

"Knowledge Guide to Tendinitis" is an invaluable resource for anyone attempting to make sense of the complex world of tendon health. Before delving into the specifics of this complex illness, the book starts with a thorough Introduction that covers the basics of tendinitis. After deciphering its essence and identifying its causes and symptoms, readers will have a solid understanding that is essential for proactive management.

An important part of the book is Anatomy and Function of Tendons, which provides a thorough examination of the fundamental structure that makes movement possible. It explains in great depth how tendons work in unison with the body, highlighting their vital role in our day-to-day actions. Through an understanding of their form and function, readers are able to appreciate the importance of maintaining tendon health.

Readers are guided through the intricate maze of Types and Causes of Tendinitis as the adventure continues, delving into the subtle nuances of this ailment.

Every aspect is carefully considered, from the root causes to the secondary effects, enabling people to recognize possible risk factors and take proactive steps to reduce them.

The chapter on Signs and Symptoms gives readers the sharp insight they need to hear the quiet murmurs of tendinitis over the clamor of everyday life. Readers are empowered to seek medical counsel when necessary by learning the critical distinction between acute and chronic signs, as well as the critical need for prompt intervention.

The journey's essential points—diagnosis and assessment—provide readers with a road plan for navigating the maze of medical examination. Through the book's demystification of diagnostic processes and emphasis on the value of a thorough examination, people are given the clarity and confidence to start their healing path.

The cornerstone of optimism is treatment options, which provide a wide range of tactics to address tendinitis.

Every option is thoroughly and carefully examined, from non-surgical therapies to the complex world of rehabilitation and recovery, making sure that readers have a full arsenal to guide them through their healing process.

The key to a future free from the confines of tendinitis is to take preventive measures, which appear as the North Star for readers. The book gives readers the tools to take control of their health by promoting proactive lifestyle changes and cultivating a culture of holistic well-being.

Rehab and Recovery is a story of resiliency that provides readers with a road map for getting their power and vitality back.

People are given the confidence to walk forward fearlessly, free from the shadow of tendinitis, by the firm support of long-term strategies and the gentle direction of rehabilitation activities.

The rich tapestry of possibilities presented by alternative therapies entices readers to investigate supplementary therapeutic paths. Every technique, from the gentle touch of massage therapy to the age-old wisdom of acupuncture, offers a different route to healing, making sure that no detail is overlooked in the pursuit of wellness.

FAQs and Common Concerns act as a compass to help readers navigate the harsh seas of doubt and uncertainty.

Through dispelling myths and providing comfort in the face of anxiety, the book shines a light on the way to a future characterized by vigor and resilience.

CHAPTER ONE

TENDONS' ANATOMY AND FUNCTION

Examining The Tendon Structure

Tendons function similarly to the strong wires that join our body's muscles to our bones. They are composed of strong, elastic tissue that is resistant to extreme strain. Think of them as the sturdy, dependable ropes that hold everything together.

If you look closely, you will notice that collagen fibers are grouped in parallel bundles to make up tendons.

Tendons are resilient and can stretch to allow for movement without rupturing because of their fibers. Consider it as a delicately woven fabric with stress resistance.

Tendon Functions In The Body

Tendons serve as the link between muscle and bone during muscular contraction, transferring force from the muscle to the bone.

Tendons act as the rope, dragging the bone along for the trip, much as in a game of tug-of-war.

Your tendon contracts each time you flex a muscle, sending the energy of the contraction to the bone and enabling efficient, painless movement.

Think of it like a smooth relay race, with you moving forward as the force (or baton, in this case) is transferred from muscle to tendon to bone.

Tendons' Function In Movement

Tendons are essential to nearly every movement you perform, ranging from the basic gait to the more intricate actions required for sports or keyboard use.

They are the unsung heroes who enable smooth motion while offering stability and support for every action.

Your tendons are working hard to make sure that your muscles and bones work together efficiently to complete the task at hand, whether you're reaching for a book on a high shelf or lifting weights at the gym.

It's similar to having a dependable group of engineers continuously adjusting your body's mechanics to keep everything functioning properly.

Tendon Health Influencing Factors

Tendons are prone to wear and strain, just like any other component of your body. Several variables, including age, degree of activity, and underlying medical issues, can affect their health.

Our tendons may become less supple and more prone to damage as we age. Similarly, engaging in demanding or repetitive tasks can overstretch tendons and raise the possibility of overuse ailments like tendinitis.

In addition, certain diseases like diabetes or arthritis can impair blood flow or induce inflammation, which can have an impact on the health of the tendons.

To preserve tendon health, it's critical to pay attention to your body's needs and adopt preventative measures like avoiding overexertion and including stretching and strengthening activities in your regimen.

Tendon Strength And Flexibility Are Important

It's essential to keep your tendons strong and flexible for both general musculoskeletal health and injury prevention. Stable and supportive tendons lower the chance of joint instability or dysfunction, whereas flexible tendons are less likely to strain or tear during physical exercise.

Regular stretching and strengthening activities will help increase the flexibility and strength of your tendons, which will enhance overall performance and lower your risk of injury. Consider it an investment in your body's structural integrity, one that will keep it robust, resilient, and able to withstand the rigors of everyday living.

CHAPTER TWO
TYPES AND ETIOLOGY OF TENDINOPATHY

Various Forms Of Tendinitis

Depending on the afflicted tendon, tendinitis can take on many forms, therefore there is no one-size-fits-all treatment for the illness.

One of the most prevalent kinds is Achilles tendinitis, which mostly affects the tendon in the rear of the ankle and is frequently brought on by overuse or an abrupt increase in physical activity.

Tennis elbow, or lateral epicondylitis as it is medically termed, is a condition that affects the tendons on the outside of the elbow and is frequently brought on by grasping or lifting repetitively.

Conversely, the tendons on the inside side of the elbow are affected by the golfer's elbow, also known as medial epicondylitis, which is frequently brought on by actions involving wrist flexion or rotation.

Finding The Root Causes

Effective prevention and treatment of tendinitis depend on an understanding of its underlying causes.

As athletes and those whose jobs require repetitive motions, like typing or physical labor, can attest, overuse or repetitive motions are frequently the main culprits.

The danger may be increased by inadequately warming up before physical activity or by not getting enough rest in between sessions.

Furthermore, without adequate training, abrupt increases in exercise length or intensity can stretch tendons, causing inflammation and tendinitis.

Comprehending Incidental Elements

Although excessive use is the main reason, tendinitis can also develop as a result of other factors.

An increased risk of injury might result from improper movement patterns or poor biomechanics, which can place excessive strain on tendons.

Unusual strains on tendons can also result from muscle imbalances, in which some muscles are developed or stronger than others.

In addition, people who already have pre-existing illnesses such as arthritis or structural anomalies may be more susceptible to tendinitis.

Lifestyle's Effect On The Development Of Tendinitis

The development of tendinitis is significantly influenced by lifestyle factors. A sedentary lifestyle can weaken tendons and muscles, rendering them more prone to damage from abrupt physical activity.

On the other hand, overusing tendons through repeated use without adequate rest and recuperation can cause inflammation and eventually result in tendinitis.

Tendinitis can be prevented by leading a balanced lifestyle that incorporates frequent exercise, good posture, and enough sleep.

Risk Elements Linked To Tendinitis

A person's risk of developing tendinitis can be raised by several risk factors. Age plays a big role because as we age, our tendons tend to lose their suppleness and become more vulnerable to injury.

A higher risk is associated with some jobs and activities that require heavy lifting or repeated motions. Tendinitis is also more common in sports like tennis, swimming, and jogging which call for repetitive actions. Furthermore, smoking, obesity, and bad posture can all harm tendons and raise the possibility of tendinitis. By being aware of these risk factors, proactive steps to avoid tendinitis and preserve the general health of your tendons can be taken.

CHAPTER THREE

INDICATES AND SYMPTOMS

Identifying Early Warning Indications

Early detection of tendinitis warning signals is essential for timely diagnosis and intervention. One typical sign is soreness or pain in the afflicted area, which is frequently made worse by pressure or movement.

The tendon may enlarge or feel warm to the touch, which are signs of inflammation. Furthermore, stiffness or a limited range of motion in the joint may indicate tendinitis early on. Keep an eye out for any adjustments to your daily schedule or level of physical activity that might be causing these symptoms.

A gradual start of discomfort during or after repetitive tasks is another inconspicuous warning indication. Should you have pain during activities that you used to undertake without any discomfort, this may be a sign that tendinitis is beginning to develop. Don't disregard these early warning signs; taking quick action can stop the illness from getting worse.

Typical Symptoms

Depending on the damaged tendon and the degree of the ailment, tendinitis can present with a variety of symptoms.

The main symptom, which usually appears at the location of the injured tendon, is pain. This pain can vary in intensity, from a dull aching to a strong stabbing feeling, especially when the tendon is being pressed or moved.

Tenderness and swelling are two more typical signs of tendinitis. The afflicted tendon may enlarge, and you may experience pressure or touch sensitivity. Because of inflammation, the area may feel warm to the touch, which is the body's immunological reaction to tissue injury.

Tendinitis occasionally results in stiffness and a restricted range of motion in the afflicted joint. Simple motions like bending or stretching the joint may become unpleasant or challenging as a result. These symptoms may intensify as tendinitis advances, making it more difficult for you to carry out daily tasks, engage in sports, and exercise.

How The Affected Area Affects The Symptoms

Depending on the particular tendon implicated and the actions that aggravate it, tendinitis can present with a variety of symptoms. For instance, pain and stiffness in the heel area are common symptoms of Achilles tendinitis, which affects the tendon in the back of the ankle. Running and jumping are two examples of activities that might aggravate these symptoms, making it challenging to participate in sports.

Tennis elbow, also known as lateral epicondylitis, is a condition that causes pain and tenderness in the area around the elbow. It damages the tendons there.

Tennis elbow can worsen when a person grips something or uses their wrists repeatedly, like when playing tennis or typing.

Similarly, the tendons on the inside of the elbow can be affected by golfer's elbow, also known as medial epicondylitis, which can result in pain and tenderness in this region.

Golfer's elbow symptoms may intensify when engaging in gripping or repetitive wrist flexion exercises like lifting weights or playing golf.

Recognising Acute Vs Chronic Tendinitis

Depending on the length of time and degree of symptoms, tendinitis can be categorized as either acute or chronic. Acute tendinitis usually appears rapidly as a result of a tendon injury or overuse.

Initial symptoms may be severe, but with rest and conservative care, they should progressively get better.

On the other hand, chronic tendinitis appears gradually and lasts for several weeks, months, or even years.

Repetitive stress or untreated acute tendinitis are common causes of it.

To properly manage chronic tendinitis, which can cause ongoing discomfort and functional restrictions, extensive treatment options are needed.

To choose the best course of action for therapy, it is critical to distinguish between acute and chronic tendinitis.

In addition to anti-inflammatory drugs and physical therapy, RICE therapy (rest, ice, compression, and elevation) may be effective in treating acute tendinitis.

More drastic measures, such as extracorporeal shock wave therapy, corticosteroid injections, or in extreme circumstances, surgical repair, may be required for chronic tendinitis.

When To Get Medical Help

For prompt diagnosis and treatment of tendinitis, it is essential to understand when to seek medical attention.

It's best to see a healthcare provider if your pain, swelling, or restricted movement persists or gets worse despite your best efforts at self-care.

It is also wise to get medical attention if your symptoms are interfering with your everyday activities, employment, or leisure activities.

Severe pain, the inability to bear weight on the injured limb, or infection-related symptoms like fever, redness, or warmth surrounding the affected area are other warning signals that call for medical treatment.

A prompt evaluation by a medical professional can assist in identifying the root cause of your symptoms and creating a suitable treatment plan to reduce discomfort and stop more issues.

Recall that effective tendinitis therapy requires early intervention. If you're unclear about the severity of your symptoms or the best course of action, don't be afraid to consult a doctor.

Personalized advice and treatment recommendations based on your unique needs and objectives can be provided by your healthcare practitioner.

CHAPTER FOUR

DIAGNOSIS AND EVALUATION

Synopsis Of Diagnostic Techniques

Healthcare providers use a range of methods to determine the underlying cause of your pain and discomfort when diagnosing tendinitis.

A comprehensive review of your medical history and any activities or behaviors that might be aggravating your symptoms is one of the first steps in this approach. This data offers insightful information about possible risk factors and directs future research.

Methods Of Physical Examination

Your healthcare professional will examine the affected area physically to look for indications of soreness, edema, and restricted range of motion. To determine the exact area of your discomfort and assess your level of pain, they could also ask you to carry out particular motions or tasks. They can detect any anomalies or regions of inflammation that can point to tendinitis by carefully palpating the tendon and the tissues around it.

Imaging Examinations For Precise Diagnosis

To confirm a diagnosis of tendinitis, imaging studies including MRIs, ultrasounds, and X-rays may be required in some circumstances. With the aid of these tests, medical practitioners can examine the interior components of the afflicted tendon and determine the degree of any inflammation or damage.

They can determine the best course of action for treating your symptoms and rule out other possible reasons by getting in-depth pictures of the affected area.

Speaking With Medical Experts

It's critical to speak with a healthcare provider if you think you might have tendinitis to receive a precise diagnosis and tailored treatment advice. To address your unique needs, your primary care physician or a specialist like an orthopedic surgeon or sports medicine physician can analyze your symptoms, conduct a thorough evaluation, and create a customized treatment plan.

The Value Of A Thorough Evaluation

To accurately diagnose tendinitis and choose the best course of treatment, a thorough evaluation is essential. Healthcare providers can better understand your condition and customize their care to match your needs by taking into account your medical history, performing a detailed physical examination, and ordering the necessary imaging tests.

This tailored approach reduces the chance of long-term problems and helps avoid recurrence in addition to guaranteeing the best possible results.

CHAPTER FIVE

OPTIONS FOR TREATMENT

Non-Surgical Methods Of Therapy

The initial line of treatment for tendinitis is frequently non-surgical techniques. Without requiring intrusive treatments, these methods aim to reduce inflammation, relieve pain, and promote healing.

The RICE method—which stands for Rest, Ice, Compression, and Elevation—is one popular strategy.

By resting the afflicted area, using ice packs to reduce inflammation, applying compression bandages for support, and elevating the injured limb to assist fluid drainage, this treatment helps minimize swelling and discomfort.

Furthermore, tendinitis-related pain and inflammation can be effectively managed with over-the-counter pain medications such as ibuprofen or naproxen.

These drugs function by lowering the body's synthesis of prostaglandins, which are molecules that cause inflammation and discomfort.

However, it's crucial to take the prescribed amount as directed and speak with a doctor, particularly if you have any underlying medical issues or are on other medications.

Another essential element of the non-surgical treatment for tendinitis is physical therapy.

A professional physical therapist can create a customized workout plan to increase flexibility, strengthen the muscles around the injured tendon, and improve joint function overall. Depending on your unique needs and capabilities, these exercises could involve range-of-motion drills, resistance training, and mild stretching.

To help with pain relief and tissue repair, additional modalities like ultrasound, heat therapy, or electrical stimulation might be applied.

Additionally, adjusting your routine might help manage the symptoms of tendinitis and avoid additional injury.

This could be avoiding activities or repetitive actions that irritate the injured tendon, modifying the ergonomics of your workspace to lessen strain, or utilizing assistive devices to lessen the tension in the injured area.

You may speed up the healing process and avoid tendinitis from happening again by adopting these lifestyle changes.

Painkillers

Medication may be used to treat persistent or severe tendinitis pain to control symptoms and enhance quality of life.

Nonsteroidal anti-inflammatory medications (NSAIDs) like aspirin, ibuprofen, or naproxen are frequently used to treat tendinitis-related pain and inflammation.

These drugs function by preventing the body from producing prostaglandins, which are molecules that increase pain and inflammation.

However because long-term use of NSAIDs might result in gastrointestinal issues or other adverse effects, it's crucial to use them carefully and under a doctor's supervision.

In certain instances, corticosteroid injections could be suggested as a temporary treatment for tendinitis symptoms.

Strong anti-inflammatory drugs are injected directly into the injured tendon using these injections, which reduces pain and swelling.

Corticosteroid injections can offer immediate relief, but because of the possibility of tendon weakening or rupturing with repeated use, they are usually administered infrequently.

To find out if corticosteroid injections are the right course of treatment for you, it's critical to go over the possible dangers and advantages with your doctor.

Methods Of Physical Treatment

Physical therapy is an essential part of the treatment of tendinitis since it helps to strengthen the surrounding muscles, reduce discomfort, and increase flexibility.

A knowledgeable physical therapist can create a customized treatment plan that fits your requirements and goals, using a range of methods to encourage healing and regain function.

Therapeutic exercise is a typical physical therapy strategy used to treat tendinitis. By strengthening and stretching the muscles that surround the injured tendon, these exercises help to improve joint stability and function and lessen discomfort and inflammation.

To help with pain relief and tissue repair, additional modalities like ultrasound, heat therapy, or electrical stimulation might be applied.

By penetrating deeply into the tissues with high-frequency sound waves, ultrasound therapy increases blood flow and facilitates the delivery of nutrients and oxygen to the wounded area.

Heat treatment, which includes paraffin baths and hot packs, can ease pain, ease stiffness in the muscles, and relax them.

On the other hand, electrical stimulation stimulates the nerves using low-level electrical currents, which lessens pain signals and encourages the contraction and relaxation of muscles.

Additionally, to increase general tissue flexibility, decrease muscle tension, and improve joint mobility, manual treatment techniques like massage and joint mobilization may be used.

Soft tissue manipulation is used in massage therapy to enhance circulation, encourage relaxation, and lessen discomfort and edema.

Joint mobilization procedures are designed to restore a normal range of motion and function by gently mobilizing stiff or restricted joints.

You can more quickly heal from tendinitis and successfully control its symptoms by using these several physical therapy strategies.

Function Of Relaxation And Activity Adjustment

Treatment for tendinitis must include both rest and activity restriction because they give the injured tendon time to recover and stop the symptoms from getting worse.

Rest is crucial during the acute stage of tendinitis to lessen discomfort and inflammation and encourage tissue repair.

To help with this, it might be necessary to temporarily refrain from high-impact exercises or repetitive motions that aggravate the condition and to allow the injured tendon enough time to heal.

Rest, though, does not equate to total immobility. To avoid stiffness and preserve joint flexibility during rest times, mild stretches and range-of-motion exercises could be suggested. Supportive devices like braces, splints, or orthotic inserts can also be used to relieve strain on the torn tendon and stabilize the affected area.

Regaining strength and function while reducing the chance of recurrence requires a cautious resumption of activities as symptoms resolve and the acute phase of tendinitis fades.

This could entail restarting activities and exercises gradually, beginning with modified or low-impact versions and escalating duration and intensity over time as tolerated.

 By collaborating with a physical therapist or another medical expert, you may create a safe and efficient return-to-activity strategy that is customized to your unique requirements and objectives.

Surgical Procedures In More Serious Situations

Surgical intervention may be required to repair or reconstruct the afflicted tendon in cases of severe tendinitis where conservative therapy has not relieved the condition or where the tendon has sustained extensive damage.

Surgery alternatives for tendinitis vary based on the location and severity of the injury as well as the specifics of the patient, including age, degree of activity, and general health.

Tendon repair, which involves surgically reattaching the injured or torn tendon to the bone using sutures or anchors, is a frequent surgical technique for tendinitis.

Usually done arthroscopically, this surgery minimizes damage to surrounding tissues and speeds up recovery by utilizing tiny incisions and specialized devices.

Tendon reconstruction or transfer may be required if the tendon is badly deteriorated or cannot be healed to give the damaged joint stability and function again.

In most cases, immobilization and rehabilitation are necessary following surgery to promote adequate tendon healing and restore strength and function.

To protect the repaired tendon, this may entail wearing a cast or splint. Next, a progressive series of physical therapy exercises is recommended to regain muscular strength, range of motion, and flexibility.

It is imperative to collaborate closely with a proficient physical therapist and adhere to a well-structured rehabilitation regimen to achieve optimal results and avoid issues like re-injury or stiffness.

CHAPTER SIX

PREVENTIVE ACTIONS

The Value Of Preventive Techniques

Treating tendinitis is far more difficult than preventing it. You can ensure your comfort and mobility by lowering your chance of having this ailment by using efficient prevention techniques. Prevention is about more than just avoiding pain; it's about preserving your quality of life and your ability to do the things you love without any obstacles.

Including Appropriate Ergonomics

In particular, ergonomics is important for people whose occupations require repetitive motions or lengthy periods of sitting or standing as a means of preventing tendinitis. Your body is positioned to put the least amount of strain on your tendons when you practice proper ergonomics. This entails utilizing ergonomic products and equipment, altering the height of your workspace, and keeping proper posture the entire day.

Warm-Up And Cool-Down Techniques That Work

You must warm up your muscles and tendons thoroughly before beginning any kind of physical activity. This lessens the chance of strain and injury by improving flexibility and boosting blood flow to the muscles. Similarly, allowing your body to gradually return to resting condition after exercise helps avoid pain and stiffness. Tendon health can be greatly enhanced by adding foam rolling, soft motions, and dynamic stretches to your warm-up and cool-down exercises.

Changes In Lifestyle To Lower Risk

Modest lifestyle adjustments can significantly lower your chance of tendinitis. Sustaining a healthy weight alleviates needless stress on your tendons, and maintaining proper hydration guarantees maximum tissue performance.

Giving up smoking can also encourage greater tissue repair and blood flow. Prioritizing rest and recuperation also reduces the chance of overuse injuries by giving your body the time it needs to heal and rejuvenate.

Encouraging General Tendon Health

Promoting general tendon health is essential to preventing tendinitis, in addition to particular preventive strategies. This entails eating a well-balanced diet high in nutrients, such as protein, vitamins C and E, and omega-3 fatty acids, that promote tissue repair and regeneration. Maintaining tendon flexibility and avoiding dehydration-related injuries also depend on getting enough water.

Furthermore, you can strengthen your tendons without overstressing them by including low-impact workouts like cycling or swimming in your program.

You can live a more active and pain-free lifestyle and considerably lower your chance of acquiring tendinitis by adopting a holistic approach to tendon health.

CHAPTER SEVEN

RESTORATION AS WELL AS RECOVERY

Knowing How The Recovery Process Works

To recover from tendinitis, one must comprehend the body's innate healing mechanism. Rest is the first important step in allowing the irritated tendons to heal.

Reducing or changing activities that worsen the disease may be part of this phase. During this phase, cold compresses or ice packs can assist reduce discomfort and inflammation.

To avoid stiffness and muscular atrophy, it's crucial to find a balance between rest and activity.

The importance of mild stretching and mobility exercises increases when the acute inflammation decreases.

The goal of these exercises is to increase the range of motion and flexibility around the injured tendon.

Physical therapy can help with this process by offering exercises and strategies that are specifically designed to address individual needs. During this stage, normal function is gradually restored, therefore consistency is essential.

Exercises for strengthening the muscles become more crucial as the healing process progresses.

These exercises work the supporting and stabilizing muscles around the injured tendon.

Using weights or bands, resistance exercise helps develop strength gradually without overstretching a tendon. To prevent further injuries, it is imperative to concentrate on using good form and technique.

It's critical to assess pain levels during the rehabilitation process and modify activities as necessary.

Pain acts as a guide, telling you when to press on and when to back off. Recovery times can vary based on the severity of the damage and each patient's reaction to treatment, so patience is crucial.

Recognizing little accomplishments along the road helps keep you motivated and moving in the direction of a full recovery.

Exercises And Methods For Rehabilitation

Exercises for rehabilitation are essential to the tendinitis recovery process.

These exercises are intended to promote healing and functional restoration while addressing certain limitations.

Exercises that increase the range of motion, such as soft stretching and joint mobilizations, aid in preserving flexibility and avoiding stiffness.

To prevent aggravating symptoms, these motions should be done at a range that doesn't cause any pain.

Rebuilding muscle endurance and strength is the main goal of strengthening workouts. Restoring balance and stability can be facilitated by addressing the nearby muscles as well as the injured tendon. For tendon rehabilitation, eccentric exercises—which entail extending the muscle under tension—are especially helpful. Over time, these exercises encourage tissue remodeling and resilience by carefully loading the tendon.

Massage and myofascial release are examples of manual treatment techniques that can be used in conjunction with exercise therapy to address soft tissue limitations and improve circulation.

These manual techniques ease tense muscles and enhance tissue integrity, which speeds up the healing process.

In addition, techniques like electrical stimulation or ultrasound can be used to improve tissue repair and reduce pain.

Functional exercises are added as the rehabilitation goes on to replicate motions and activities from everyday life. These workouts aid in the transition from recovery to resumed every day or sports-related activities. For example, strengthening neuromuscular control, balance, and proprioception exercises can improve coordination and reduce the risk of re-injury.

Returning Gradually To The Activity Guidelines

To reduce the chance of recurrence, tendinitis recovery after rehabilitation calls for a methodical and gradual return to activities. Achieving a balance between providing the tendon with enough challenge to encourage adaptability and preventing overstress that can result in re-injury is crucial.

This process is facilitated by a graded return-to-activity plan, which progressively increases duration and intensity over time.

Low-impact exercises that don't exacerbate the tendon are the main emphasis of the initial phase.

This could involve minor strength training in addition to mild cardiovascular exercises like swimming or walking. During this stage, diligent observation of symptoms enables any necessary adjustments to avoid setbacks.

Activities can be progressively more complex and intense as tolerance grows. This could be adding exercises unique to your sport or progressively going back to playing competitive or recreational sports to the fullest. It's critical to pay attention to the body's signals of pain or discomfort and to heed them, modifying the rate of advancement as necessary.

Proper warm-up and cool-down routines are crucial to the process of returning to action because they prime the body for exercise and speed up recovery. Static stretching and foam rolling can help with post-exercise recovery and lessen muscle discomfort, while dynamic stretching and mobility exercises help the muscles and tendons get ready for action.

Handling Obstacles During Rehabilitation

Setbacks are a normal component of the tendinitis rehabilitation process and should be seen as transient obstacles rather than immovable barriers.

Overcoming obstacles requires perseverance, fortitude, and a proactive attitude. The first thing to do when experiencing a setback is to determine any possible causes or contributing elements, such as misuse, bad biomechanics, or insufficient recuperation.

To address the underlying causes of the setback, modifications to the rehabilitation program or activity level might be necessary.

This could entail adding more rest days, temporarily lowering or changing activities, or going over certain elements of the rehabilitation plan again, including exercise choice or intensity.

During this period, seeking advice and support from a physical therapist or other healthcare expert can be very beneficial.

Managing setbacks involves not just attending to bodily issues but also to mental and emotional health. Overcoming obstacles more skillfully can be accomplished by keeping a positive mindset, establishing reasonable expectations, and engaging in self-care practices. It's critical to appreciate little accomplishments along the road and to concentrate on progress rather than perfection.

Long-Term Methods Of Recurrence Prevention

Adopting long-term methods to address underlying risk factors and promote overall tendon health is necessary to prevent tendinitis from recurring.

This could entail making adjustments to work or training habits, enhancing movement patterns and biomechanics, and adding sensible rest and recuperation techniques into everyday schedules.

By dispersing the stress across several muscle groups and movement patterns, cross-training and diversifying your activities can help lower your risk of overuse injuries. Enhancing general resilience and lowering the chance of injury can also be accomplished by including strength and conditioning exercises that focus on specific muscle imbalances and deficiencies.

Choosing the right equipment and technique is crucial, especially when participating in sports or other activities that require high-impact or repetitive movements.

Over time, the risk of injury can be decreased and excessive strain on the tendons can be minimized by using the right footwear, equipment, and technique.

Preventing recurrence also requires routine tendon health maintenance and monitoring.

This can include planning regular check-ins with a medical practitioner or physical therapist for assessment and guidance, as well as including periodic rest periods or deload weeks into training regimens.

Furthermore, being aware of the early warning indicators of tendinitis, such as localized soreness or stiffness, enables timely treatment and stops the condition from getting worse.

CHAPTER EIGHT

OPTIONAL THERAPIES

Investigating alternative therapies can provide a comprehensive approach to pain management and recovery when it comes to tendinitis. These therapies can frequently offer extra support and relief in addition to conventional treatments.

Examining Complementary Medicine

There are several different techniques outside of traditional medicine that are used as complementary treatments for tendinitis.

These treatments are meant to improve the body's inherent ability to heal while also reducing symptoms.

Chiropractic therapy is a well-liked alternative that focuses on joint manipulation and spinal alignment to enhance general musculoskeletal health.

Furthermore, methods like physiotherapy and osteopathy might help injured tendons regain their range of motion and functionality.

Acupuncture's Function In Pain Management

Tiny needles are inserted into certain bodily locations during the ancient Chinese art of acupuncture to encourage the flow of qi and aid in healing.

Although the precise mechanism underlying acupuncture's efficacious treatment of tendinitis remains incompletely comprehended, numerous patients report notable alleviation of pain and enhanced range of motion after receiving the therapy.

The natural painkillers produced by the body, endorphins, can be released, blood circulation increased, and inflammation reduced by acupuncture.

Advantages Of Therapeutic Massage

Massage treatment targets soft tissues and promotes relaxation as a non-invasive way to manage the symptoms of tendinitis.

Numerous methods, including myofascial release, deep tissue massage, and Swedish massage, can help remove muscle tension, enhance blood flow, and lessen the discomfort and stiffness brought on by tendinitis.

Furthermore, massage treatment can improve damaged joints' range of motion and flexibility, which can speed up the healing process.

Using Supports And Braces

As a typical adjunct in the treatment of tendinitis, braces, and supports give wounded tendons stability and defense. By immobilizing the injured area, these devices lessen tension and stop additional injuries from occurring during regular activities or exercise. Different braces and supports—from wrist splints for wrist tendinitis to knee braces for patellar tendinitis—may be advised depending on the location and degree of tendinitis.

Possibility Of Herbal Remedies Being Effective

For generations, people have turned to herbal medicines to treat a wide range of illnesses, including tendinitis and other musculoskeletal disorders. Some herbs have analgesic and anti-inflammatory qualities that can help lessen tendinitis-related pain and swelling. Among the herbs that are frequently used for tendinitis are arnica, Boswellia, ginger, and turmeric. These herbs can be administered locally to the affected area as lotions or ointments, or taken orally as supplements.

Beyond standard medical measures, adding alternative therapies to your tendinitis treatment strategy might provide further relief and support. To guarantee the safety and efficacy of any new therapy, you must speak with a healthcare provider beforehand, especially if you have underlying medical conditions or are on medication. You can manage tendinitis and improve your general health by investigating complementary therapies including acupuncture,
massage therapy, and herbal remedies.

CHAPTER NINE

COMMON QUESTIONS AND ANSWERS

Dispelling Myths Regarding Tendinitis

Misunderstood frequently, tendinitis is not solely related to aging or misuse. Anybody can be impacted by it, regardless of age or degree of exercise. One widespread misunderstanding is that the best course of action is usually relaxation. In addition to rest, strengthening the injured tendon and averting further flare-ups require suitable exercise and physical therapy.

Another common misperception is that tendinitis will go away on its own. While some cases might get better with time, many others need specialized care to cure completely and avoid long-term problems. Ignoring tendinitis can result in the condition getting worse and possibly causing the tendon long-term harm.

Handling The Fear And Anxiety Caused By The Illness

Managing tendinitis can be mentally exhausting, particularly if it makes regular tasks or hobbies difficult. It's normal to have anxiety due to the unpredictability of the healing process and the possibility of obstacles. Some of these anxieties can be reduced, though, if you are aware of the illness and adhere to a regimented treatment plan.

The anxiety brought on by tendinitis can also be reduced by engaging in relaxation exercises like deep breathing or meditation. Keeping up to date on the condition and talking with medical professionals about any concerns you may have can also offer comfort and direction as you work towards recovery.

Faqs Regarding Changes In Lifestyle

It might be necessary to make some lifestyle adjustments to cope with tendinitis, but it doesn't imply giving up on your favorite pastimes. Achieving a balance between physical exercise and rest is crucial. Don't overdo it, but also keep within your physical limitations.

Purchasing supportive shoes or ergonomic keyboards, for example, can also assist reduce the tension that goes on strained tendons when performing daily duties. Furthermore, sustaining a healthy lifestyle that includes balanced eating and frequent exercise might aid in the general healing process and avert relapses.

Resolving Surgery-Related Fears

Surgery is usually only advised as a last option for tendinitis when all other therapies have failed to relieve the condition.

Because they are worried about the pain, recuperation period, and possible complications, many people are afraid of surgery.

On the other hand, less invasive operations with shorter recovery times and a lower risk of complications have been made possible by advances in surgical techniques.

It's critical to address any worries or inquiries you may have regarding surgery with a medical professional to comprehend the advantages and risks unique to your circumstances.

Sources Of Continued Assistance And Knowledge

To effectively manage tendinitis, support and information are essential. Online resources, such as reliable medical forums and websites, can offer insightful commentary and guidance from others who have faced the same difficulties.

There may be opportunities to connect with people who are going through similar challenges with tendinitis through local support groups or community organizations. Furthermore, medical professionals such as orthopedic specialists and physical therapists can provide tailored advice and assistance during your recuperation process.

www.ingramcontent.com/pod-product-compliance
Lightning Source LLC
Chambersburg PA
CBHW071842210526
45479CB00001B/245